Prolotherapy: The Truth About Prolotherapy

A Complete Beginner's Guide to Cure Lower Back Pain, Tendinitis, and Osteoarthritis

D1728558

presentation of the information is without contract or any type of guarantee assurance.

The trademarks that are used are without any consent, and the publication of the trademark is without permission or backing by the trademark owner. All trademarks and brands within this book are for clarifying purposes only and are owned by the owners themselves, not affiliated with this document.

Table Of Contents

Introduction

If you are suffering from joint problems such as lower back pain, tendinitis, or osteoarthritis, among others, you are not alone. There are millions out there who are enduring pain from joint problems, and most of them settle for simply managing such pain. Although managing the pain can be your best option for chronic pain brought about by neuropathic illnesses and cancer, it is not the same for chronic musculoskeletal pain. More than sixty years ago, a cure known as "prolotherapy" was developed to relieve and/or treat joint problems.

Prolotherapy is becoming more popular nowadays, as many people are searching for alternative treatments to surgery for alleviating lower back pain, tendinitis, and osteoarthritis. In the 1940's, only a few doctors specialized in this treatment. However, through the years, more and more people shared their success stories about being cured from prolotherapy techniques.

Given that joint pain can impair an individual, the search for relief is almost immediate, as is the consumption of various pain medications. However, when joint pains worsen, common knowledge tells patients to undergo some sort of surgery. In fact, in some cases, patients may be directed to hip or knee joint replacements.

More often than not, sufferers of different joint pains avoid techniques or procedures that require a long time for recovery, yet the procedure may not be completely successful. For instance, some joint replacements are only good for a few years and may require another joint replacement after a while. Some patients are also concerned about recalls or class action lawsuits against joint replacements, which are often advertised on television.

Today, many people are opting to go with prolotherapy treatments, as they are said to have less risks and provide a quicker process of healing as compared to most other treatment methods. This is because prolotherapy capitalizes on the natural ability of the body to heal itself. The weakening of tendons and ligaments often causes joint pains. For those unaware, these are the structures that keep the bones and muscles together. The weakening of these structures puts stress on the bones' sensitive areas.

During a prolotherapy treatment, a patient is injected with a mild irritant directed into the affected area. The immune response of the body to the inflammation leads to the blood flow increase in the affected area, as well as the rebuilding of the tissues. Consequently, there will be stronger and thicker tendons and ligaments. In addition, the stress is removed from the bone over time. The patient will then notice an increase in mobility as the pain subsides. Although a prolotherapy treatment does not work instantly, it requires less recovery time than most surgeries. Moreover, the improvement on the patient can be drastic.

In this short, concise book, you will gain a thorough understanding of prolotherapy. Chapter 1 discusses what prolotherapy is in a more in-depth manner. Chapter 2 discusses the history of this treatment method. Chapter 3 discusses the effects of prolotherapy on different joint pains. Chapter 4 discusses the advantages and disadvantages of the treatment. Chapter 5 discusses prolotherapy compared to other treatments. Lastly, Chapter 6 discusses the future of prolotherapy in the always-evolving world of medicine.

We hope you are able to learn a thing or two!

Chapter 1:

What is Prolotherapy?

Prolotherapy involves a technique focused on injection treatments designed to induce healing. It causes a temporary, mild inflammation in the affected area. This inflammation sets off the fibroblasts to the injection site, which change precursors into mature collagen, reinforcing the connective tissue.

Direct exposure of fibroblasts to either endogenous or exogenous growth factors results in new cell growth, as well as collagen disposition. The inflammation involved in prolotherapy produces secondary elevation of growth factors. This means that through prolotherapy's inflammatory stimulus, the level of growth factors is elevated in order to restart or initiate a new repair sequence of connective tissue that was aborted prematurely or never started at all. After conducting prolotherapy injections, the ligament is thickened, the tendon is strengthened, and the tendinosseous junction is enlarged.

More often than not, prolotherapy is used for joint problems or musculoskeletal injuries, or pains that persist for at least eight weeks. As mentioned previously, it works by elevating the efficiency or levels of growth factor, causing repair or production of new tissues. Prolotherapy is usually used years after the initial joint problem originally transpired, provided that the individual is in a healthy condition. Given that prolotherapy is meant to repair painful joint areas, it is considered a long-term solution.

Types of Prolotherapy and the Science Behind Them:

Dextrose Prolotherapy

Dextrose prolotherapy is the original form of prolotherapy, which originated in the 1930's. This type makes use of saline (salt water), concentrated dextrose (sugar water), or other natural substances as an irritant for stimulating a moderate inflammation in the affected area. Dextrose prolotherapy elevates the efficiency or levels of growth factor in order to repair tissue or reduce or eliminate the pain caused by joint problems.

Physicians across the globe who practice the use of dextrose prolotherapy have proven the efficiency of the treatment in alleviating various musculoskeletal conditions. These include back and neck pain, joint laxity and instability, ligament sprains, tennis elbow, plantar fasciitis, ankle pain, tendinopathies, and shoulder and knee pain, among others.

Dextrose prolotherapy is often referred to as simply *prolotherapy,* as it is the method's original form.

Platelet Rich Plasma (PRP) Prolotherapy

This type also involves a process of injection, which is also meant to induce healing. *PRP* is referred to as autologous blood that has platelet concentrations higher than baseline levels. It is said to have no less than seven growth factors. PRP cell ratios have 94% platelet concentration, compared to normal blood cells that only have 6% platelet concentration. Platelets consist of a number of cytokines, proteins, and other bioactive factors that all encourage and regulate the basic aspects of the natural healing process.

There are circulating platelets that secrete growth factors, such as vascular endothelial growth factor in angiogenesis, insulin-like growth factor – 1 (for mediation of growth and repair of skeletal muscle), fibroblast growth factor (for the proliferation of angiogenesis and myoblasts), platelet-derived growth factor (for stimulating angiogenesis and cell replication), and others.

When platelet concentration is increased through PRP, the possibility of enhanced healing is increased as well. When the platelets are activated, they signal distant repair cells to address the site of injury. These repair cells include adult stem cells. As the volume of platelets is increased, the subsequent flow process of repair and stem cells is also increased. Given that the concentrated platelets are held in a small plasma volume, the three plasma proteins, namely vitronectin, fibrin, and fibronectin, take part in the repair process. While dextrose prolotherapy can be compared to merely planting seeds, PRP is similar to planting seeds with fertilizer.

Biocellular Prolotherapy

Although both dextrose prolotherapy and PRP are meant to induce healing, they rely on the body to have sufficient local repair cells, specifically in the affected area or injury site. In the event that the joint area is injured and inflamed chronically for an extended period of time, cellular depletion transpires. This translates to not having enough repair stem cells at the injury site because they are already used up.

When there is cellular depletion, local repair stem cells will no longer be available, or those remaining will be used up during several treatments of either dextrose prolotherapy or PRP. Consequently, *biocellular prolotherapy* is done to acquire good repair cells from the adipose/fat tissue or bone marrow. Apart from not supplementing additives, the cells are not manipulated. In addition, the cells acquired are from the same patient and will also be returned to the patient in the same day and procedure.

The adipose tissue and the bone marrow are said to have sufficient adult stem cells that can be used as the stimulant for the injury site. In some studies, researchers claim that every tissue has stem cells. However, the adipose tissue and bone marrow are the main sources of the body in which extra repair cells can be acquired as needed.

The formula used in biocellular prolotherapy is autologous tissue, which is derived from adipose or fat tissue, bone marrow, and/or PRP. When the fat is the formula, the method is referred to as *lipoaspirate prolotherapy*, which involves a method of liposuction for extracting the fat. On the other hand, when the formula is the bone marrow, the method is referred to as *bone marrow prolotherapy*. Both of these methods are forms of biocellular prolotherapy.

Cells Derived from the Bone Marrow

Researchers studied the use of adult Mesenchymal Stem Cells (MSCs) in tendon repair in as early as 1998. The researchers concluded that using implanted adult stem cells brought to tendon defects could ameliorate the structure, biomechanics, and the function of the tendon significantly after injury.

In 1995, MSCs were considered to be safe for human utilization. Once the researchers had established the safety of MSCs, further research was conducted. The ability to direct onto a target and repair areas of tissue injury is one of the most prominent observations regarding these repair cells. The stem cell potency of a patient may be depleted due to specific degenerative diseases such as osteoarthritis. This is because there is a reduction in the proliferative ability and capacity to differentiate.

During the following years, researchers continuously studied the bone marrow. In their studies, one consistent fact remained: the bone marrow contained adult stem cells. One of the most important elements in the efficiency of cells derived from the bone marrow is the latter's concentration. There are also available FDA approved devices that allow the bone marrow's concentration into Bone Marrow Aspirate Concentrate (BMAC). BMAC contains accessory cells and mesenchymal stem cells, which support angiogenesis and vasculogenesis through the production of growth factors and cytokines. An increasing amount of evidence shows that the combination of PRP and BMAC is equivalent to autologous bone grafting.

In addition, BMAC is also deemed to be safe as well as effective in treating tibial nonunion, Jones fracture, metatarsal nonunion, osteochondral defect repair, osteonecrosis of the hip, and limb ischemia. In India, a five-year study using BMAC for non-reconstructable critical limb ischemia was conducted. Based on the results, BMAC provided 90% amputation-free survival and 90% reduction of pain.

Stem or Stromal Cells Derived from Adipose

According to numerous studies, the human adipose tissue is an abundant source of adult stem cells. Furthermore, its cell population has extensive proliferative capacity, as well as the ability to discern into multiple lineages of cells. While many people do not mind if they give up a little fat, many are willing to go an extra mile to eliminate fat through undergoing liposuction procedures. The fat that is eliminated contains useable volumes of adipose tissue. Stem or stromal cells that are derived from adipose can develop into tendons, ligaments, cartilage, muscle, fat, or bone.

For many years, fat grafting has been a part of cosmetic procedures. Furthermore, this lipoaspirate is also used in musculoskeletal medicine, whether or not there is PRP. This is because lipoaspirate creates a bioactive scaffold or gel matrix that holds the inflammatory stimulant in a joint area. Stem or stromal cells that are derived from adipose are similar to bone marrow cells, although they are not identical.

Stem or stromal cells that are derived from adipose are used with BMAC and/or PRP for treating various musculoskeletal and vascular problems. Researchers claim that the PRP fat graft is induced for the cell type that is surrounding it. For instance, if the PRP fat graft is placed with muscle cells, then it will develop into muscle. Given that fat harvesting is simpler that bone marrow aspiration, the utilization of autologous adipose tissue is becoming more popular in the office setting. In addition, the production of stem cells from adipose tissue is higher than with bone marrow by about 500 to 1,000 times.

Chapter 2:

History of Prolotherapy

The history of prolotherapy dates back to ancient times, with its earliest known form used by the Egyptians for treating crippled animals. During this time, the method of prolotherapy involved the use of hot iron cautery. On the other hand, prolotherapy was first used in humans circa 400 BC. It was said that Hippocrates found a way to repair a dislocated shoulder by using a hot poker in the axilla, or armpit.

In 1835, the father of prolotherapy, Dr. Alfred A.L.M. Velpeau, injected an iodine solution into a patient in order to treat a hernia. Around 1880, Dr. Rene Leriche injected ligaments that contained procaine, which demonstrated a pattern or pain from an injury and ligament laxity. The primary condition treated by prolotherapy from the 1830's to the early

1920's was the hernia. In 1926, the American Society of Herniologists was created to carry out procedures for hernias, hemorrhoids, and varicose veins. It was also the first organization to use prolotherapy.

1930's to 1950's

The origin of modern-day prolotherapy was brought about by the innovation of an osteopathic physician and surgeon, Dr. Earl Gedney. It was in the early 1930's when Gedney's thumb was caught in a surgical suite door. This incident stretched the joint of his thumb and caused severe pain. Gedney's colleagues told him that no treatment could be done for his condition. Consequently, his condition would also lead to the end of his career.

However, Dr. Gedney pursued research and became resolved to becoming "his own doctor." He was aware that some members of the American Society of Herniologists were using irritating solutions to treat hernias. Consequently, Gedney used this knowledge to inject his impaired thumb.

In 1937, Gedney published the first known article, "The Hypermobile Joint," which was about injection therapy, then known as *sclerotherapy*. This article provided two case reports of a patient with low back pain and another with knee pain. Both patients were treated successfully with the injection therapy. The article also provided a preliminary protocol.

On February 1938, Gedney wrote another paper that included an outline of the technique. He presented the paper in the meeting of the Osteopathic Clinical Society of Philadelphia.

The 1930's were a remarkable time for injection therapy. This is because a number of researchers conducted their extensive histologic research on the technique. These researchers include Matson, White, Rice, Harris, Manoil, and Biskind. They all discerned that collagen was being restored at the injury site. In addition, they also claimed that specific and consistent cellular events transpired, accounting the positive results from the injection therapy.

All throughout the 1940's and into the mid 1950's there was an increase in the publication of articles concerning the use of prolotherapy outside of the treatment for hernias. Researchers discovered that the injection therapy could be used for the musculoskeletal system at large. In the mid 1950's, Dr. George Hackett, a general surgeon in the United States, called the injection therapy as "proliferation" through his observation that the abundant growth of new tissue was a result of the conjugation of bone and ligament. Later, Hackett renamed "proliferation" as prolotherapy, in which *prolo* refers to growth or proliferation of tissue.

By the end of the 1950's, Hackett demonstrated his research at various national conferences. He provided an in-depth understanding regarding the concept wherein enthesopathies and ligament laxity were the fundamental pathophysiology of chronic pain patterns.

1980's

During the 1980's, while other formulas were deemed efficient, the solutions that were used primarily were dextrose-based. Across the globe, physicians practiced prolotherapy, as it was viewed effective in relieving and/or treating various musculoskeletal conditions, such as ligament sprains, tendinopathies, back/neck pain, ankle pain, plantar fasciitis, and joint instability and laxity.

In 1983, Liu, along with other researchers, showed that collagen was produced at injury sites in which 5% morrhuate sodium was injected. In 1985, Maynard and his colleagues demonstrated that the biochemical and morphologic effects of morrhuate prompted the sequence of injury repair, specifically in ligaments and tendons. Klein, Ongley, and their colleagues carried out double-blind experiments that have significantly contributed through the scientific method with substantial outcomes, presenting the efficacy of prolotherapy as compared to controls.

Other researchers have also made important contributions in terms of the advancement of prolotherapy, including Pomeroy, Dorman, Mooney, Faber, Schultz, Leedy, Montgomery, and Hauser.

Prolotherapy Organizations

Through the years, various organizations have joined as one of the founding of the American Osteopathic Academy of Sclerotherapy (AOAS). In 1961, Dr. Hackett and Dr. Hemwall created the Prolotherapy Association, while Dr. Pomeroy founded the American Association of Orthopedic Medicine (AAOM). In 1996, the AOAS, which was also the parent chapter of the AAOM, was restructured, and therefore the American College of Osteopathic Pain Management and Scelerotherapy (ACOPMS) was created.

Today, the American Osteopathic Association of Prolotherapy Regenerative Medicine serves as the most prominent organization in the field of injection therapy.

Chapter 3:

The Effects of Prolotherapy

The effects of prolotherapy may vary depending on the joint pain or condition. For instance, it has a different effect on lower back pain, tendinitis and osteoarthritis. It also has a unique effect on sports-related pain or injury.

Prolotherapy and Lower Back Pain

When it comes to lower back pain, the substance is injected into the soft tissue during the prolotherapy procedure. This causes a mild inflammation in the affected area, which causes natural healing. The effects of prolotherapy for back pain include: increased strength of the tendon, ligament, or joint capsule, reduction or elimination of back pain, improved or return to normal function, and reduced recurrence of injury to the affected/treated site.

Prolotherapy and Tendinitis

The ideal first-line treatment for tendinitis is prolotherapy. This is because the procedure induces the repair of the affected tendon and strengthens any lax or weakened ligaments that surround the joint. On the other hand, if the tendons are consistently stressed and tendonitis does not improve, the tendon will eventually degenerate and lead to tendinosis. In this case, comprehensive prolotherapy should be conducted. This involves treating all of the areas in which the tendon is attached to bone, as well as the weakened tissue structures.

Prolotherapy and Osteoarthritis

Based on the findings, prolotherapy improves standard care of osteoarthritis in specific patients. It can be used in clinical practice, given that the procedure is uncomplicated. In fact, prolotherapy is carried out in the outpatient setting and does not call for ultrasound guidance.

Side Effects of Prolotherapy

Some patients who have received prolotherapy injections report mild side effects after the procedure. These include irritation and mild pain at the affected area(s), which usually lasts up to 72 hours. There are also reports of mild bleeding and numbness at the injection area. However, pain from prolotherapy is only temporary and can be relieved by taking acetaminophen. In few cases, opioid medications are suggested, specifically for patients with pain refractory.

Other side effects of prolotherapy include: bruising in the injection area, swelling, increased pain, joint effusion, stiffness, puncture of the lung, infection, nerve injury, spinal headache, and tendon/ligament injury.

Because prolotherapy causes mild inflammation, a patient will notice some pain, bruising, swelling, and stiffness in the injection area after the procedure is carried out. In general, these side effects can last up to seven days. It is only very seldom that these side effects last longer than a week. On the other hand, lingering pain can also be a sign of healing after receiving prolotherapy treatment because it works through inflammation. If there is severe pain, especially when accompanied by fever, then the patient should call or consult the physician who carried out the procedure. There should not be excessive pain after prolotherapy in any circumstance.

Meanwhile, the most serious side effect of prolotherapy is the risk of infection. If so, the infection usually occurs in the skin. Generally, this type of infection is treated with an oral antibiotic. If there is a blood or joint infection, then intravenous antibiotics are usually needed.

The risks involved with undergoing a prolotherapy procedure are usually related to the actual technique. As such, it is necessary to look for a clinic that is well equipped not only with knowledge but also experience.

Chapter 4:

Pros and Cons of Prolotherapy

Depending on the individual and his or her circumstances, there are various reasons to try prolotherapy. However, it is advisable to take a look at some of its pros and cons prior to proceeding with this procedure.

The Pros

One of the most well known advantages of prolotherapy is its capability to rapidly increase the production of collagen and cartilage in the body. Collagen and cartilage are responsible for activating the capability of the immune system to heal itself.

Another advantage of prolotherapy is its capability to treat discomfort associated with hand/foot pain, lower back pain, leg pain, ankle pain, knee pain, shoulder pain, hip pain, and even moderate to severe migraines. Apart from managing and treating discomfort, prolotherapy also fortifies and restores joints and the soft tissues in the body.

Given that prolotherapy increases the production of collagen in the body, it then strengthens the body's skeletal structure. This is because of the increase in connective tissue production as a result of the increase in collagen production.

Prolotherapy can work in all areas of the body. Because of this, it is widely accepted and practiced globally by many pain treatment specialists who have proven its efficiency in minimizing or eliminating pain, even if they are highly specialized professionals.

Prolotherapy is known as the leading alternative to alleviate or eliminate pain and, at the same time, provide numerous other benefits. For instance, it can help a patient restore his or her well-being prior to experiencing excruciating pain.

Finally, prolotherapy promotes healthy cartilage, which in turn decreases the possibility of cartilage-related disorders such as arthritis and rheumatism.

The Cons

As much as there are advantages, prolotherapy also has a few disadvantages. For one, it is a medical treatment/procedure that makes use of invasive technique that brings about various risks. Although not all patients may feel or experience side effects, one of the most common risks of prolotherapy is mild to moderate pain during and after treatment.

It is ironic that it can relieve and remove pain when it can also introduce a new kind of pain after its execution. Some patients may experience pain for a couple of minutes or hours after the treatment, which is primarily due to the invasive technique.

As previously mentioned, patients may differ in how their body reacts to the treatment. The worst side effect can be an infection in the affected area or even in the blood or joint. In some rare cases, a few patients were reported to suffer from a mild stroke after the treatment was given to them. On the other hand, this is a very rare circumstance given that patients are checked for other health complications prior to receiving prolotherapy treatments.

Chapter 5:

Prolotherapy vs. Prolozone

More often than not, prolotherapy is being compared to other joint pain treatments. One of the most common medical treatments being equated with prolotherapy is prolozone. Both are regenerative medicine treatments that are used for relieving and/or treating joint problems, such as lower back pain, tendinitis, and osteoarthritis.

Formula

There are a number of similarities and differences between prolotherapy and prolozone. However, both procedures involve non-surgical injections. On the other hand, the difference of the two lies in the formula they use. For instance, prolotherapy makes use of a sugar solution, or dextrose mixture, coupled with an anesthetic known as lidocaine. The formula also consists of a small amount of vitamin B12 for promoting healing.

Meanwhile, prolozone makes use of an anesthetic known as procaine and a B vitamin mixture, which consists of B12, multi-B vitamins, and folic acid. Its formula also includes sugar water or dextrose, a homeopathic solution, and sodium bicarbonate. After making this solution, it is injected with ozone gas.

Number of Injections

The number of individual injections is usually less with prolozone, depending on the area to be treated. This is because the solution used in prolozone treatment affects a larger area as a result of the ozone gas injection, as compared to the solution for prolotherapy.

Severity of Pain Experienced

Both procedures may bring a small amount of pain to a patient, given that they involve piercing of the skin. However, when it comes to post-injection pain, it is said that prolotherapy provides a patient with a greater amount of pain than prolozone. This is because prolotherapy makes use of a larger concentration of dextrose, along with related inflammatory effects. Some doctors make use of a topical cooling spray to provide relief from the discomfort of the needle piercing the skin.

Frequency of Procedure and Number of Visits

During the initial prolotherapy treatments, a patient may need to go back two to four weeks apart, in order to have the procedure performed, while prolozone treatments take one to two weeks between visits. The duration between treatments gradually increases when the condition of the patient improves.

When it comes to the number of visits, it varies for both treatments as well as the condition of the patient. Both prolotherapy and prolozone require one to four visits for a mild condition, five to eight visits for a moderate condition, and more than eight visits for a severe condition. On the other hand, both treatments should manifest improvement after a few sessions in order to warrant continued visits.

Cost of Treatment and Time Spent

The cost of prolotherapy and prolozone is almost the same, ranging from $150 to $400, depending on the condition of the patient and the area being treated. The amount of time that each procedure demands for an individual treatment or session is longer with prolozone as compared with prolotherapy.

Recovery Rate

The recovery rate of these two treatments varies as well. Recovery is based on the response of the patient, so some patients respond better to prolotherapy while others respond better to prolozone. More often than not, when a patient does not respond as expected to one of these regenerative medicine treatments, the other treatment is recommended.

Expected Results

Both treatments have the same expected result: to regenerate collagen in order to strengthen and/or rebuild tendons, ligaments, and cartilage. However, they differ in their mechanism and how the outcome is achieved. Prolotherapy makes use of more dextrose, which results in a stronger inflammatory response. On the other hand, prolozone makes use of procaine and ozone gas, which results in regenerative effects.

The advantages of having both treatments as an option is that patients have a choice regarding which treatment they would prefer, and in the case that they are not able to respond to the first treatment, there is an alternative available.

In this comparison, the cost, rate of recovery, number of visits, and the expected outcome are almost the same for both regenerative medicine treatments. They only differ in the solutions or formulas used, the frequency of visits, and the number of individual injections for every visit.

Most importantly, prolotherapy and prolozone both have proven track records in regards to being successful treatments. In addition, both are widely used across the globe to help patients alleviate a wide range   of   joint   problems.

Chapter 6:

The Future of Prolotherapy

Apart from the traditional prolotherapy treatment, platelet rich plasma (PRP) and stem cells are also available for stimulating the process of healing musculoskeletal injuries and pain moderation.

The expansion of the use of PRP into orthopedics transpired in the early 2000's. The reason for this expansion was to increase healing in bone fractures and grafts. Due to its success, PRP is now encouraged for use in sports medicine, specifically for repairing connective tissue. In 2006, researchers Pavelko and Mishra, who were both associated with Stanford University, published the first study that supported the use of platelet rich plasma for chronic tendon problems. Based on the study, a 93% pain reduction was achieved in two years of follow-up.

In 2008, Hines Ward, the wide receiver for the Pittsburgh Steelers, received PRP treatment for a knee medial collateral ligament sprain. Ward claimed that if not for PRP, then he would not have played for the Steelers and helped the team win the Super Bowl XLII. Other high profile athletes also received PRP treatment for various sports-related injuries, such as golfer, Tiger Woods, and Los Angeles Dodgers closer, Takashi Saito.

The demand and accessibility of PRP for more portable and affordable machines have grown as the use of the treatment has also increased worldwide. In fact, several models are now available, allowing physicians to produce PRP from a small sample of the blood of a patient. Machines are becoming more affordable and various companies now offer complimentary machines with a minimum purchase of their preparation kits.

On the other hand, the marketed PRP devices/machines are not universally the same. For instance, they differ in the quantity of blood required, viability, platelet concentration, and number of spin cycles. One of the first PRP devices that were approved by the FDA was from Harvest Technologies. Its system makes use of a floating shelf technology that allows the preservation of platelet viability until it is used.

Today, in spite of the controversies and skepticism regarding the treatment, PRP is still gaining wider acceptance in the world of sports. This is partially because there are continuous studies and research for the validation of PRP treatment for knee osteoarthritis, chronic elbow tendinosis, jumpers knee, rotator cuff tendinopathy, ligament and tendon injuries, degenerative knee cartilage, muscle strain and tears, and plantar fasciitis.

Conclusion

Thank you for reading this! We hope this short, concise book was able to teach you a thing or two about prolotherapy.

Now that you understand the important factors regarding prolotherapy, you can decide if you want to try it, or if you can inform your friends who ask you about it. Plus, a little addition to your knowledge doesn't hurt, right? Our world is becoming increasingly interested in the use of alternative treatment methods, in hopes to enhance the human experience on Earth.

If you've learned anything from this book, please take the time to share your thoughts by sending me a personal message, or even posting a review on Amazon. It would be greatly appreciated and I try my best to get back to every message!

Thank you and good luck in your journey!

Printed in Poland
by Amazon Fulfillment
Poland Sp. z o.o., Wrocław

86526282R10040